Depression and Sexual Function

Depression and Sexual Function

David S Baldwin
Senior Lecturer in Psychiatry
Faculty of Medicine, Health and Biological Sciences
University of Southampton
Southampton, UK

Sally C Thomas
Research Fellow
University Department of Psychiatry
Royal South Hants Hospital
Southampton, UK

MARTIN DUNITZ

Acknowledgements

We would like to thank Chris Thompson, Nik Martin, Marie Carter and Pam Stacey of the University Department of Psychiatry in Southampton for their encouragement, assistance and support. Further thanks are due to our publishers Martin and Ruth Dunitz, to Martin Blenkinsop of Bristol Myers Squibb Pharmaceuticals Ltd. and Dinesh Bhugra of the Institute of Psychiatry. We are forever indebted to Sally Baldwin and Tom Sulkin for their encouragement and forbearance during the preparation of the book.

August 1996

First published in the United Kingdom
in 1997 by
Martin Dunitz Ltd
The Livery House
7– 9 Pratt Street
London NW1 0AE

A CIP record for this book is available from the British Library.

ISBN 1-85317-360-6

Printed and bound in Spain by Cayfosa

Contents

Introduction

"Sexual expression is an essential component of human relationships, and in itself may promote quality of life and a sense of physical, psychological and social well-being."

This statement, included within the report of *The National Survey of Sexual Attitudes and Lifestyles* (Wellings et al, 1994) emphasizes the importance of satisfactory sexual relationships to overall health. Although sexual health has been identified as a target for medical intervention by the Department of Health in the UK, and despite the seemingly greater openness to discussion of sexual matters, little detail is known of the sexual behaviour of the general population. When the essential nature of sexual relations to continuing existence is considered, this lack of reliable information is surprising.

Whilst the findings of the *National Survey* describe many aspects of the sexual behaviour of a largely healthy community sample within the UK, much less is known of the sexual health and function of patients suffering from physical illness or from mental health problems. Although many psychiatrists take a special interest in the management of patients with sexual problems, the interrelationships of mental disorder and sexual behaviour have not been studied extensively (Bancroft, 1989).

The studies which have been performed show that the sexual health of people suffering from depression is often poor. In some, this is clearly due to the effects of depressive illness on the individual. In others, it results from the deleterious consequences of depression on interpersonal relationships. However, in many depressed patients, this loss of sexual health either arises from or is worsened by the sexual side effects of psychotropic drugs (Baldwin, 1996).

Many patients who are taking antidepressant drugs will experience sexual difficulties. However, before ascribing these problems to a particular drug, many other possible causes of sexual dysfunction need to be considered. A range of factors should be evaluated, including the features of the depressive disorder itself, the nature of any co-morbid psychiatric or physical illness, and the use of other drug treatments.

Antidepressant drugs can have adverse effects on any part of the normal sexual response. The spectrum of drug-induced sexual dysfunction includes the reduction of sexual desire, the impairment of physiological arousal, and the disturbance of orgasm. These adverse effects result from a variety of mechanisms.

Within the central nervous system, non-specific effects such as sedation can produce a decrease in sexual interest, whereas specific actions on particular neurotransmitters can lead to impairment of sexual function. Actions within the autonomic and peripheral nervous systems may also lead to sexual difficulties. Furthermore, many drugs have either direct or indirect effects on the hormones involved in the regulation of sexual activity.

The management of a patient who complains of sexual difficulties should start with a detailed assessment of the reported problem, and an investigation of the possible causes. Many forms of treatment are possible, including psychological, behavioural and surgical approaches. The range of pharmacological strategies which may prove helpful include the withdrawal of medication, the use of so-called 'drug holidays', changing from the implicated drug to another one, and the use of adjunctive treatments (Baldwin, 1996).

Sexual function and dysfunction

Classification of sexual problems

Sexual problems are common both in the general population and in clinical practice. They can cause much distress to individuals and to their partners, but many people who are troubled by sexual difficulties feel too embarrassed to seek medical advice. It is particularly important that doctors know how to take a clear and sensitive psychosexual history. Of course, this is helped by a knowledge of normal sexual physiology, and by a familiarity with the more common sexual problems.

Sexual problems can be divided into three broad groups. The first group, the **sexual dysfunctions**, involve disturbances of the normal mechanisms of sexual desire, arousal and orgasm, which can all be affected by a range of physical and psychological factors. The second group, the **gender identity disorders**, include both transvestism and trans-sexuality. Finally the third group, known as the **paraphilias**, are characterized by sexual arousal that is associated with unusual or unacceptable objects or activities, for example paedophilia, in which the sexual attraction is towards children (Webster, 1996).

This book is concerned with the assessment and management of sexual dysfunction in patients with depression. Therefore, no further mention will be made of the gender identity disorders or the paraphilias, except to note that a small minority of depressed patients can develop an unusual variation in sexual interest, often in an attempt to relieve anxiety and reduce feelings of inner tension. More typically, depression is associated with the various forms of sexual dysfunction.

The World Health Organisation ICD-10 classification of sexual dysfunction is shown in Table 1, and the American Psychiatric Association DSM-IV classification is shown in Table 2. The two classificatory systems have many more similarities than differences (Potts and Bhugra, 1995). The DSM-IV has no category for excessive sexual drive, but separates the sexes when coding the disorders of arousal and orgasm, and it includes two additional categories of sexual dysfunction — that due to a general medical condition, and substance-induced sexual dysfunction. The DSM-IV also allows a further classification of the sexual dysfunctions according to their duration, to the situation in which they occur, and to the relative contribution of organic and psychological factors.

ICD-10 classification of sexual dysfunction	
Disorders of desire	Lack or loss of sexual desire Sexual aversion and lack of sexual enjoyment Excessive sexual drive
Disorders of arousal	Failure of genital response
Disorders of orgasm	Orgasmic dysfunction Premature ejaculation
Disorders of sexual pain	Nonorganic vaginismus Nonorganic dyspareunia
Other disorders	Other sexual dysfunction, not caused by organic disorder Unspecified dysfunction not caused by organic disorder *Source: World Health Organization (1992)*

Table 1

DSM-IV classification of sexual dysfunction	
Disorders of desire	Hypoactive sexual desire disorder Sexual aversion disorder
Disorders of arousal	Female sexual arousal disorder Male erectile disorder
Disorders of orgasm	Female orgasmic disorder Male orgasmic disorder Premature ejaculation
Disorders of sexual pain	Dyspareunia (not due to a general medical condition) Vaginismus (not due to a general medical condition)
Other disorders	Sexual dysfunction due to a general medical condition Substance-induced sexual dysfunction Sexual dysfunction not otherwise specified *Source*: *American Psychiatric Association (1994)*

Table 2

The sexual response cycle

By convention the sexual response cycle is regarded as having four phases (Figure 1). This classification was first proposed by Masters and Johnson in the 1960s, and developed by Kaplan in the subsequent decade. A full description of the normal sexual response cycle is available in textbooks of sexual medicine (e.g., Bancroft, 1989).

The first phase of the cycle ('**desire**') comprises sexual interest and drive. Sexual desire is probably the part of the sexual response that is the most difficult to conceptualize, being essentially an experiential rather than a neurophysiological phenomenon. It has three dimensions, which interact not only with each other, but also with cultural, psychological and hormonal influences (Bancroft, 1989):

Cognitive	—	Sexual thoughts and imagery
Affective	—	Mood and other emotional states
Physiological	—	Central arousability (transmission of and response to sexual cues)

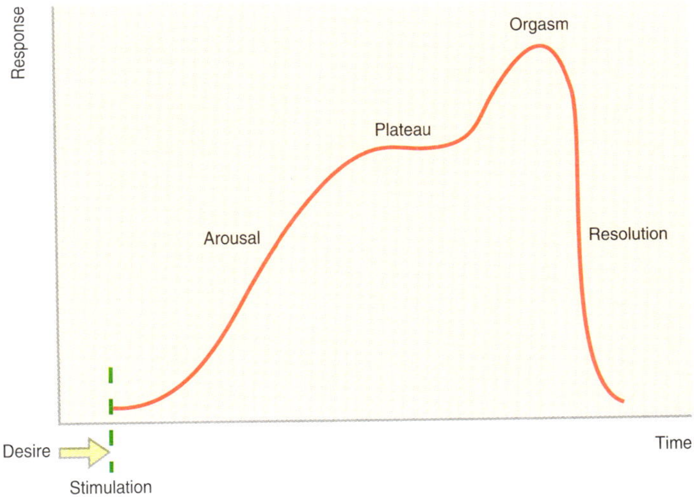

Figure 1
Human sexual response.

The second phase in the sexual response cycle ('**arousal**') is characterized in men by tumescence and erection of the penis, and in women by vaginal lubrication and 'ballooning' of the vaginal walls. These genital changes are accompanied by other manifestations of arousal such as raised blood pressure, an increased heart rate and altered body temperature.

Many aspects of the physiology of penile erection remain unclear. What is generally agreed is that stiffness depends on filling of the erectile tissues in the corpora cavernosa with blood, rigidity arising from the effects of this increased pressure being contained within the tough fibrous tunica albuginea. Other changes during arousal in men include thickening and contraction of the scrotum.

Sexual arousal in women is more extensive and complex. Genital changes include engorgement of the corpora cavernosa of the clitoris, and of the venous plexus around the lower part of the vagina and the erectile bulbs of the vestibule. Further changes include moistening of the vaginal epithelium and an increase in size of the upper two-thirds of the vagina.

The third phase ('**orgasm**') involves emission and ejaculation in men, and orgasm, which can be multiple, in women. Many aspects of orgasm are subjective — for example, the sense of loss of control or altered consciousness — and are therefore rather difficult to define and measure. Other aspects of orgasm are more amenable to study — for example, the range of objective changes in the genitalia, changes in skeletal muscle tone, and cardiovascular and respiratory responses.

The final phase of the sexual response cycle is known as '**resolution**'. In this stage, there is a fairly rapid return of the physiological manifestations of arousal and vasocongestion to normal, with an accompanying sense of calm. Without orgasm, these changes take longer to resolve, and in women can result in an uncomfortable congestion of the pelvic organs. In men resolution is usually followed by a refractory period during which no response occurs to further sexual stimulation. By contrast, women may be able to experience multiple orgasms within a short period.

Dysfunction can occur in any phase of the sexual response cycle. For example, decreased libido and hypersexuality are two types of desire phase dysfunction. Problems that occur in the arousal phase include erectile failure or a lack of vaginal lubrication. Orgasmic phase problems include premature or inhibited ejaculation in men, and anorgasmia in women. Within an individual a problem in one area is often associated with difficulties in another, and it is not uncommon for both partners within a sexual relationship to be troubled by sexual dysfunction.

Plan for the assessment of sexual dysfunction

The assessment of a patient who complains of sexual difficulties whilst taking a psychotropic drug should involve the detailed evaluation of a range of factors (Gitlin, 1994; Baldwin, 1995) (Table 3).

Assessment of sexual dysfunction
Premorbid sexual function
Primary psychiatric disorder
Co-morbid psychiatric disorder
Co-morbid physical illness
Psychotropic medication
Concomitant medication
Source: Gitlin (1994); Baldwin (1995)

Table 3

Specific enquiries should be made into each stage of the sexual response. It seems sensible for doctors to develop a series of questions that can be asked easily without causing undue embarrassment to either the patient or the doctor. These questions will relate to the problems of decreased sexual desire, difficulties in achieving or maintaining erection or vaginal lubrication, and to problems in achieving orgasm.

Having identified the exact nature of the sexual problem, it is then necessary to assess whether the difficulties change with time, or vary according to circumstance. Tactful enquiries should be made into whether there have been any changes in the quality of any intimate relationships or in the number of sexual partners.

The process of assessment should continue with enquiries about the pattern of sexual activity even before the patient became unwell, as sexual problems are commonplace in the general population. It is then necessary to assess the degree of sexual interest and function present whilst the patient was depressed, but before they started treatment. Further steps in evaluation include an assessment of the nature of any co-morbid psychiatric or physical illness.

Patients should then be questioned about their consumption of psychotropic drugs and use of other classes of medication, whether these were prescribed by a doctor, or obtained 'over the counter' from a chemist. If it seems appropriate, the patient should be asked about the use of alcohol and 'recreational' drugs, as these may have untoward effects on sexual function.

Finally, whenever possible, and with the consent of the patient, attempt to speak to any sexual partner, to assess and discuss the impact of the difficulties on the sexual and overall relationship. Many depressed patients and their partners will be relieved to learn that their doctor has recognized the sexual problem, and that help may be available.

Causes of sexual dysfunction

Epidemiology of sexual problems

Unfortunately, there have been rather few epidemiological investigations that are of sufficient rigour to allow an accurate estimate of the true prevalence of sexual difficulties within the general population. This relative lack of 'normative' data should be remembered when considering the incidence of sexual dysfunction in patients suffering from depressive illness.

The investigations which have been performed tend to suggest that sexual problems are common in the general population. For example, in a study of 100 'happily married' couples:

- 14% of women and 15% of men stated that they were either 'not very' or 'not at all' satisfied with their sexual relationship
- 40% of men reported erectile or ejaculatory problems
- 63% of women described problems with arousal or orgasm

Sexual dissatisfaction and dysfunction appears common even in seemingly happy relationships (Frank et al, 1978).

Figures such as these are not unrepresentative of the findings of other studies. In an analysis of the results of 22 surveys of the general population (Nathan, 1986), sexual disorders were found to be common:

- Inhibited sexual desire was considered to be present in up to 15% of men and 35% of women
- 10–20% of men had inhibited sexual excitement
- 35% of men were or had been troubled by premature ejaculation
- Inhibited orgasm was found in 5% of men and up to 30% of women

There have been few studies of the incidence of sexual difficulties amongst patients in primary care settings. However, the results of an investigation of men and women attending their general practitioner for non-sexual problems (Golombok et al, 1984) suggest that sexual dysfunction is common:

- 20% of women described difficulty in becoming sexually aroused
- 7% were anorgasmic, 17% with their partner
- 7% of men described transient erectile problems
- 20% of men reported premature ejaculation

In spite of these difficulties, 97% of the men and 77% of the women said that they were satisfied with their sexual relationship.

Although sexual problems are common in both men and women, a male patient who develops sexual difficulties is more likely to seek and receive medical attention (Shen and Sata, 1983). This may be because male sexual anatomy and physiology are such that problems can be described relatively easily. Studies indicate that men may be more willing than women to describe sexual problems to psychiatrists, women being prepared to report problems only after direct questioning (Harrison et al, 1986; Shen and Sata, 1990).

Depression and sexual function

Depressive illness is often associated with impairment of a range of aspects of sexual function. Depressed patients complain of a general reduction in interest, the loss of energy, and a pervasive inability to gain pleasure. Depression should therefore be expected to lead to sexual difficulties. In addition, depression is also linked to reduced self esteem, and to irritability and social withdrawal, all of which can cause problems in forming and maintaining intimate relationships.

Many depressed patients describe a reduction in their sexual interest and activity. This decline is usually associated with other depressive symptoms, including 'biological' symptoms such as weight loss, reduced energy and disturbed sleep. The results of a Finnish epidemiological survey suggest that a change in sexual interest is an indicator of depression in all groups, other than in women older than 70 years. For older women in that study, a change in libido appeared to be a normal part of ageing (Kivela and Pahkala, 1988).

In certain investigations, a minority of depressed patients describe an increase, rather than a reduction in sexual activity. This increase may be due to an anxious search for reassurance and intimacy, rather than being a reflection of a genuine increase in sexual desire (Matthew and Weinman, 1982).

Although loss of sexual desire is probably the most common sexual difficulty experienced by patients with depression, other forms of dysfunction are also common. For example, in a comparative study of the sexual function of depressed patients and that of age- and sex- matched controls, erectile dysfunction was present in up to 35% of depressed men, but in none of the control subjects. Furthermore, premature or delayed ejaculation were described by 38% and 47% of the depressed patients, compared to 0% and 6% of the controls, respectively (Matthew and Weinman, 1982).

Loss of sexual interest may be the presenting complaint of some patients. On closer questioning, many will be found to be suffering from depression. Even if not currently depressed, patients with low sexual desire have often suffered from depression in their past (Schreiner-Engel and Schiavi, 1986). As the loss of sexual desire may have been a feature of earlier episodes of depression, it makes sense to follow up patients who complain of this problem, particularly when there is a history of depressive illness.

Of course, many patients will simultaneously have both a psychiatric disorder and a disorder of sexual function. For example, in an early study, sexual and marital difficulties were reported by 25% of patients attending a psychiatry outpatient clinic, and sexual or marital therapy was considered to be suitable in approximately half of the patients (Swan and Wilson, 1979). A more recent study indicated that sexual dysfunction was present in 36% of outpatients with severe affective illness, compared to 49% of outpatients with schizophrenia, and 13% of patients receiving treatment for a range of dermatological disorders (Kockott and Pfeiffer, 1996). Finally, an investigation of the extent of co-morbidity of sexual problems and mental disorder among patients with a primary diagnosis of sexual dysfunction found that a dual diagnosis was present in 30% of men and 31% of women. In addition to the sexual dysfunction, affective illness was present in 16% of men and 30% of women (Fagan et al, 1988).

Public attitudes to depression and sexual health

The relative importance of sexual health to patients with depression can be surmised by considering the results of a study conducted by the MORI Health Research Unit for LMB Public Relations, on behalf of the pharmaceutical company Bristol Myers Squibb Pharmaceuticals Ltd.

In this investigation, 6143 interviews were conducted in the UK between May and June, 1995. Of the total survey sample, a group of 1140 (17%) subjects were, or had previously been, 'depressed':

- 891 (15%) had been depressed according to a modified version of the Research Diagnostic Criteria for depression (Spitzer et al, 1978)
- 458 subjects (7%) had been diagnosed as suffering from depression by their doctor. Clearly, a number of respondents with depression had not sought medical attention
- Of the total study sample, 466 (7%) stated that they had been prescribed 'antidepressants', 6% stated that they had been prescribed 'sleeping tablets', and 5% reported that they had been given 'tranquillizers'

When asked about the importance to overall health of a list of factors, 70% of the total sample and 75% of the depressed group thought that 'having a good sex life' was either very or fairly important. This compares to figures of 98% for feeling fit and healthy, 95% for sleeping well, 94% for having a normal appetite, and 90% for getting regular exercise. Although these figures suggest that satisfactory sexual relations are considered to be somewhat less important than other 'lifestyle factors', they do indicate that sexual satisfaction is important to people suffering from depression, as normal controls and depressed subjects did not differ in this respect.

The survey suggests that sexual problems are probably less important than other aspects of the depressive syndrome in determining consultation with a doctor, for example when compared to feeling suicidal, sleeping poorly, or being low in mood. Only 3% of the total sample, and 2% of the 'depressed' group, thought that loss of sexual interest would be the factor most likely to prompt a visit to their general practitioner.

When asked about the symptoms they would most want cured, 8% of the total sample stated that loss of sexual interest would be the difficulty they most wanted relieved, this figure being the same in the 'depressed' group. Again, as a problem, loss of sexual interest was considered to be less in need of resolution than either feeling low or sleeping poorly.

As loss of sexual interest is a component of the depressive syndrome, it could be thought that a response to treatment with antidepressant drugs should be linked to improvements in sexual function. The results of the MORI survey suggest that this is not necessarily the case. Although 51% of the sub-sample who had been prescribed antidepressants stated that they either felt less depressed or no longer felt depressed with treatment, only 1% described an increased interest in sex whilst having treatment. Adverse effects of antidepressants on sexual function were more common, as 8% of the group stated that treatment caused either a loss of interest in sex, or other forms of sexual dissatisfaction.

Substance abuse and sexual dysfunction

Many depressed patients drink alcohol to excess, often to relieve unbearable states of tension. Although alcohol possesses some anxiolytic properties, it is a central nervous system depressant and excessive or prolonged consumption of alcohol can act as a maintaining factor in depressive illness. In addition, depressive syndromes are common in alcohol dependent patients, and can act as a stimulus to continued drinking.

Similarly, depressive syndromes are often associated with substance abuse, particularly in younger patients. As the incidence of depression in young people appears to be increasing, the problem of co-morbid depression and drug abuse or dependence is likely to become more common. This section describes some of the untoward effects of alcohol and recreational drugs on sexual function.

Alcohol

The effects of alcohol on sexual function are variable, probably because people have differing expectations of the impact of alcohol upon sexuality. In both men and women, beliefs about the sexual effects of alcohol can lead to increased drinking and can influence sexual activity whilst intoxicated. The results of an early survey of normal volunteers suggested that 45% of men and 68% of women felt that alcohol enhanced sexual enjoyment, whereas 42% of men and 21% of women felt that it decreased sexual pleasure (Athanasiou et al, 1970). Further investigations tend to indicate that alcohol has inhibitory effects on sexual activity, greater impairment being reported with increasing consumption.

The acute effects of alcohol on sexual arousal are probably mediated by spinal reflexes. At levels greater than 40 mg/dl, alcohol has direct pharmacological effects upon sexual performance. Acute intoxication with alcohol causes a transient decrease in plasma testosterone, probably due to toxic effects of ethanol and its metabolites on the testes. Alcohol does not appear to affect the pituitary-gonadal hormones in women.

Long-term abuse of alcohol can affect sexual function in a variety of ways. For example, peripheral neuropathy which can impair sensory input, and damage to autonomic nerves which can affect the physiology of arousal and orgasm. In men, prolonged alcohol abuse can decrease testosterone levels, raise the level of sex-hormone-binding globulins, and increase oestrogen levels. These effects are probably mediated via the hypothalamo-pituitary-gonadal system, rather than simply being a consequence of alcohol-induced liver disease (Huws and Sampson, 1993).

Alcohol dependence syndrome is often thought to be associated with sexual dysfunction. Uncontrolled studies suggest that erectile dysfunction is common, being reported by 44–59% of male 'alcoholics'. A controlled study of male alcoholics revealed that the patient group had a greater incidence of erectile failure, and reported less sexual satisfaction (Whalley, 1978). This finding was supported by the results of a further investigation, in which 84% of 44 men admitted to an outpatient alcohol treatment programme were found to have either erectile dysfunction or ejaculatory failure (Mandell and Miller, 1983). The high prevalence of sexual problems in alcohol dependent patients does not appear to be restricted to men. In a survey of the alcohol consumption of women living in the USA, moderate drinkers of alcohol had lower levels of sexual dysfunction than either heavy drinkers or light or abstinent drinkers (Klassen and Wilsnack, 1986).

In certain people, alcohol is used as a tranquillizer to blunt emotional pain that arises from difficult relationships and sexual problems. In others, becoming intoxicated with alcohol can be a way of avoiding sexual intercourse. Relationship difficulties that result from alcoholism may themselves lead to increased drinking, which can then worsen the existing sexual and interpersonal problems.

Cannabis

Although use of cannabis is often thought to enhance sexual pleasure, most recent research seems to suggest that it has little effect upon sexual performance. Regular users of cannabis report that it can lead to delayed ejaculation, and to an increase in sexual satisfaction. The reported beneficial effects of cannabis upon sexual function may be largely due to heightened expectations, or to a general sense of euphoria, relaxation and enhanced sensory awareness. Heavy use of cannabis may be associated with sexual dysfunction, but again no clear conclusions can be drawn (Huws and Sampson, 1993).

Opiates

Regular use of opiates — both prescribed and non-prescribed — is associated with reduced sexual interest, erectile failure and delayed ejaculation. Many regular users have endocrine abnormalities, arising from an uncertain mechanism. In women users, menstrual abnormalities including amenorrhoea are common. Testosterone levels tend to be low in diamorphine dependence, and are consistently low in patients undergoing maintenance treatment with methadone. Acute opiate use increases prolactin levels, and a few studies have shown that prolonged use may also cause hyperprolactinaemia (Huws and Sampson, 1993).

Stimulants

The effects of psychostimulant drugs such as amphetamines, cocaine, 'Ecstasy', and amyl nitrite on sexual function are far from clear. For example, studies of regular amphetamine users suggest that some subjects describe improvements in sexual behaviour, whilst others report delayed ejaculation. In a study of cocaine use in massage parlours, the male clients felt that cocaine increased their sexual desire but made erection and ejaculation more difficult, whereas the female prostitutes found that the main effect of cocaine was to keep them awake and suppress negative cognitions! (Wesson, 1982). Prolonged use of cocaine is often associated with the loss of sexual desire.

Media reports that Ecstasy is a 'love drug' do not appear to be supported by the findings of research, for although it can be associated with a sense of 'closeness' to other people, sexual effects are not often mentioned. Amyl nitrite is used widely in the homosexual community, and has a range of effects on sexual function including the reduction of sexual inhibition, delays in ejaculation and relaxation of the anal sphincter (Huws and Sampson, 1993).

Physical illness and sexual difficulties

Community surveys

As part of the *National Survey of Sexual Attitudes and Lifestyles* (Wellings et al, 1994), a sample of 18,876 people aged 16–59 years was questioned about their perceived health, and the presence of any disability that restricted work or leisure activities. The subjects were also asked whether or not they suffered from any long term medical condition that needed regular treatment or checkups, or whether they had in the preceding 5 years any illness or accident that had affected their health for at least 3 months. In addition, the sample gave details of their average alcohol consumption, cigarette smoking, and their height and weight (Wadsworth and Johnson, 1994).

There was only a limited relationship between perceived physical health and sexual behaviour. The frequency of heterosexual intercourse was only weakly related to perceived overall health. Although less frequent intercourse was associated with poor health, much of this association appeared to be due to the fact that poorer health itself is linked to older age. In general, perceived physical health seems to have little influence on sexual lifestyle.

As regards cigarette smoking, there was a striking trend for heavier smoking to be associated both with increasing numbers of sexual partners and with a greater number of sexual encounters within a given period. This pattern of association was also seen for alcohol consumption; the proportion of moderate and heavy drinkers of alcohol rose in line with increases in the frequency of sexual encounters and the number of sexual partners.

These findings seem to confirm the notion that there is a relationship between a number of risk-taking behaviours. However, there was an inverse relationship between sexual behaviour and obesity, greater body mass index (weight / height^2) being found to be linked to a reduced number of sexual partners.

Clinical settings

Sexual dysfunction seems to be common in patients referred to general medical outpatient clinics. For example, a survey of 1180 male medical outpatients found that 34% had erectile problems (Slag et al, 1983). In another study, approximately 50% of 228 patients interviewed or responding to a questionnaire described sexual problems. For many patients, the sexual problems were related to their medical illness. Interestingly, 91% of patients thought that it was appropriate for a doctor to take a sexual history, contradicting the belief held by some doctors that patients will be upset by being questioned about sensitive matters (Ende et al, 1984).

Many medical conditions are associated with both depression and sexual dysfunction (Table 4). These conditions include

Physical ill health which can affect sexual behaviour

System	Example
Neurological	Cerebrovascular accident, spinal injuries, multiple sclerosis
Vascular	Myocardial infarction, peripheral vascular disease, arteriolar damage
Endocrine	Pituitary lesions, diabetes mellitus, reduced testosterone levels
Gastrointestinal	Ileostomy
Urogenital	Pelvic disease, trauma, cancer
Cancer	Breast, testis, leukaemia

Source: Crowe (1995)

Table 4

neurological disorders such as multiple sclerosis, peripheral and autonomic neuropathy, stroke and spinal cord injuries, and cardiovascular problems including myocardial ischaemia and peripheral vascular disease. Endocrine disorders that may have adverse effects on sexual function include diabetes mellitus, hypothyroidism and hypopituitarism. Many other conditions may impair sexual health — often due to a combination of the direct effects of the illness itself (for example, malignancy), the disability which can result from the condition, and the adverse effects of prescribed medication (Bancroft, 1989).

Sexual problems are also common amongst patients attending gynaecology outpatient clinics. Studies performed in the USA indicate that sexual problems are reported by up to 30% of patients, and sexual dysfunction is described by around 20% of patients (Levine and Yost, 1976). A survey of Dutch gynaecologists indicated that sexual problems were the presenting complaint in approximately 7% of their patients, the most common of these difficulties being loss of sexual desire and dyspareunia (Frenken and van Tol, 1987).

These studies indicate that sexual function and health may be affected adversely by a range of medical conditions. However, the results of the *National Survey* indicate that physical health and sexual behaviour are not necessarily closely related. Many severely ill patients enjoy satisfactory sexual relations, and many people in good physical health suffer from sexual dysfunction. Therefore, sexual dysfunction in a depressed patient who also has a medical condition should be ascribed to the physical illness only after careful consideration of other possible causes.

Investigation of sexual dysfunction

Further assessment of a patient with sexual dysfunction can include a number of rather complex investigations (Schiavi,

1992), including measures of nocturnal penile tumescence, arterial waveform analysis and peripheral nerve conduction tests, but these are used only infrequently and are best performed in specialized clinic settings (Bancroft, 1989). Some of these investigations are listed in Table 5.

Investigation of sexual dysfunction
Nocturnal penile tumescence
Strain gauge monitoring
Erectile response to erotic stimuli
Penile blood flow during erection
Intracavernosal injections of smooth muscle relaxants
Pudendal nerve latency time
Sacral evoked response
Sources: Bancroft (1989); Schiavi (1992)

Table 5

There has been little objective research into the sexual function of depressed patients. A number of studies have attempted to evaluate the pattern of nocturnal penile tumescence and rigidity in depressed men, compared to that seen in normal controls. Although early studies suggested that there was a complete absence of penile tumescence in states of severe depression in elderly patients, more recent work indicates that in younger depressed men there is only a relative decrease, and that this is not associated with the severity of depression, but rather with the presence of the endogenous sub-type of depressive illness (Bancroft, 1989).

Usually, sexual problems result from a combination of psychological and 'organic' factors. Although physical examination or specialized investigations may reveal the presence of an identifiable 'lesion', this should not be assumed to provide a full explanation for the sexual dysfunction, and the role of psychological and interpersonal factors should always be considered.

Adverse effects of drugs on sexual function

Neurotransmitters and sexual behaviour

For a behaviour that is so clearly vital to human existence, it is surprising that so many aspects of the physiological basis of the human sexual response remain unclear. Furthermore, although research in animal models can provide some insight into human sexual behaviour, the findings of such studies are often not applicable to other species. However, it is clear that male and female sexual behaviour is affected by a number of neurotransmitters, some of which have complex actions (Table 6). The following account is only a brief description of the sexual pharmacology of some of the neurotransmitters: further details can be found elsewhere (Riley et al, 1993; Segraves, 1989).

In general terms, **dopamine** seems to facilitate sexual activity, probably through actions within the central nervous system. It increases sexual behaviour in experimental male animals, this effect being blocked by central but not peripheral dopamine antagonists. The effects of dopamine on female sexual behaviour in animal models vary, according to whether the animal is in a receptive or non-receptive state (Wilson, 1993). In clinical settings, dopamine agonists such as bromocriptine can increase sexual interest and activity. By contrast, dopamine antagonists such as the antipsychotic drugs are often linked to the development of sexual dysfunction.

Neurotransmitters with effects on sexual behaviour
Dopamine
Noradrenaline
Serotonin
Acetylcholine
GABA
Oxytocin
Arg-vasopressin
Angiotensin II
Gonadotrophin-releasing hormone
Substance P
Neuropeptide Y
Cholecystokinin-8
Source: Segraves (1989); Wilson (1993)

Table 6

Like dopamine, **noradrenaline** has a significant role in sexual behaviour, but has both central and peripheral actions. In animal models of male sexual behaviour, enhancing central noradrenergic activity often results in increased sexual arousal. However, the peripheral actions of noradrenaline can impair sexual performance, through the inhibition of penile reflexes. Any effect on copulatory behaviour is probably indirect (Wilson, 1993).

The role of **serotonin** (5-hydroxytryptamine, 5-HT) in sexual behaviour is not fully understood. Studies in experimental animals have produced rather inconsistent findings, but suggest that 5-HT has different effects in females and males (Wilson, 1993). In general, increased transmission within central serotonergic pathways usually produces a reduction in sexual arousal and activity. In animal models, these inhibitory actions are mediated by 5-HT_2 receptors. Peripheral serotonergic fibres probably inhibit penile sensation and ejaculation.

These findings correspond with the observation that in man, sexual dysfunction associated with serotonin re-uptake inhibitors can be reversed by 5-HT_2 antagonists. The stimulatory effects on sexual behaviour that are sometimes seen with agents acting on other 5-HT receptors, such as buspirone which acts on the 5-HT_{1a} autoreceptor sub-type, are probably due to inhibition of the release of serotonin.

Acetylcholine may have only a limited role in regulating sexual activity. In male animal models, it reduces arousal but also reduces the threshold for ejaculation. Acetylcholine may have indirect effects, as optimal sexual function probably depends on a balance of adrenergic and cholinergic effects. Cholinergic agonists such as neostigmine and bethanechol can be helpful in reversing the erectile dysfunction that is seen with certain antidepressant drugs (Segraves, 1993).

Gamma aminobutyric acid (GABA) seems to have inhibitory effects on sexual behaviour, independent of its effects on motor activity (Wilson, 1993). In animal models, benzodiazepine agonists such as diazepam, which exert their effects through actions on GABA, reduce male sexual activity, whereas benzodiazepine antagonists reverse the effects of agonists, but themselves have no effect on sexual behaviour.

Adverse effects of antidepressant drugs on sexual function

Many psychotropic drugs have untoward effects on sexual function. Within the central nervous system, non-specific effects such as sedation can produce a decrease in sexual interest, and specific actions on certain neurotransmitters can lead to impairment of sexual function. Actions within the autonomic nervous system may also lead to sexual difficulties. Furthermore, many drugs have either direct or indirect effects on hormones that are involved in the regulation of sexual activity (Table 7).

Adverse effects of psychotropic drugs on sexual function
Nonspecific effects on the central nervous system
Specific effects on neurotransmitters within the central nervous system
Specific effects on neurotransmitters within the autonomic nervous system
Direct effects on hormonal activity
Indirect effects on the regulation of hormones
Sources: Segraves (1989); Gitlin (1994)

Table 7

Data derived from the results of placebo-controlled clinical trials show that antidepressant drugs are often associated with the development of sexual dysfunction. However, the true incidence of sexual difficulties is likely to be even greater than that reported, for a number of reasons (Baldwin, 1995).

Sexual problems are discussed in clinical settings only rarely. Many patients do not feel comfortable when discussing sexual problems, and will therefore not mention any difficulties to their doctor. Although some patients will report sexual problems when completing a questionnaire, others will describe sexual dysfunction only after direct questioning by the doctor. Furthermore, the variation in the description of clinical terms and the absence of a generally accepted standardized schedule for eliciting sexual difficulties can also lead to inconsistencies when reporting sexual problems.

As such, it seems likely that only the most troublesome sexual side-effects are reported, there being a greater number of other problems that only come to light with direct questioning. For example, systematic enquiries in a sample of 60 patients, prescribed a number of different antidepressant drugs including imipramine, fluoxetine, trazodone and desipramine found that sexual dysfunction during treatment occurred in 43.3% of patients. The presence of sexual dysfunction was not related to diagnosis, the antidepressant that was prescribed, or the presence of anticholinergic side effects (Balon et al, 1993).

Tricyclic antidepressants

The sexual side effects of tricyclic antidepressants (TCAs) have not been investigated to any great extent. Until recently, most of the data were derived from single case reports or small case series. TCAs have been implicated in the development of most forms of sexual dysfunction, including decreased sexual interest, erectile failure, impaired ejaculation and impaired orgasm. Erectile difficulties and problems with ejaculation have been described in patients taking amitriptyline, imipramine, clomipramine, desipramine, nortriptyline and protryptyline. Anorgasmia has been reported with imipramine, clomipramine, desipramine, nortriptyline and doxepin. The relative incidence of these problems with differing drugs has not been reliably determined (Segraves, 1993; Baldwin, 1996).

Sexual dysfunction may be especially common with the TCA clomipramine. In a placebo-controlled study of the treatment of patients with obsessive compulsive disorder, 33% of those receiving clomipramine spontaneously reported sexual problems. Furthermore, when asked to complete a questionnaire, 66% of clomipramine-treated patients described sexual difficulties, this figure increasing to 95% after direct questioning. By contrast, none of the patients treated with placebo reported sexual dysfunction (Monteiro et al, 1987) (Table 8).

Monoamine oxidase inhibitors

As with the tricyclic drugs, most of the reports of sexual dysfunction with monoamine oxidase inhibitors (MAOIs) are limited to single case reports or small case series. Like TCAs, MAOIs have

Placebo-controlled study of clomipramine in obsessive compulsive disorder

Sexual dysfunction	Clomipramine n = 24	Placebo n = 9
Spontaneous reports by patient	8	0
Self-completed questionnaires	16	0
Specific enquiries by physician	22	0

Source: Monteiro (1987)

Table 8

been associated with the development of most forms of sexual dysfunction, including decreased sexual interest, erectile failure, impaired ejaculation and impaired orgasm (Baldwin, 1995).

Although there are reports of increased sexual desire with isocarboxazid, its effects, and those of pargyline, on other aspects of sexual function are largely unknown. By contrast, phenelzine has been linked to impairments of erection, ejaculation and orgasm. There are few published reports of erectile dysfunction or ejaculatory failure with tranylcypromine. Preliminary findings suggest that moclobemide, a reversible inhibitor of monoamine oxidase type A, may have fewer adverse effects on sexual function than the conventional non-selective MAOIs (Philipp et al, 1993).

Sexual difficulties may be rather more common with MAOIs than with TCAs. In a comparative study of phenelzine, imipramine and placebo, sexual dysfunction was reported by 80% of men and 57% of women taking phenelzine, compared with figures of 50% and 27% for imipramine, and 8% and 16% for patients taking placebo. Accurate evaluation of the presence of

Relative incidence of sexual dysfunction with TCAs and MAOIs: Placebo controlled study of imipramine and phenelzine in depression

	Imipramine	Phenelzine	Placebo
Sexual dysfunction: men	50%	80%	8%
Sexual dysfunction: women	27%	57%	16%

Source: Harrison (1986)

Table 9

sexual dysfunction in the depressed women was especially dependent upon the use of specific enquiries (Harrison et al, 1986) (Table 9).

Selective serotonin re-uptake inhibitors

As with TCAs and MAOIs, the selective serotonin re-uptake inhibitors (SSRIs) have been implicated in the development of sexual dysfunction in a number of case reports and case series, as well as in the results of controlled clinical trials. During the course of development of the SSRIs, most studies seemed to show that they had a relatively low incidence of sexual dysfunction. However, these findings have had to be revised upward as the drugs have entered widespread use in clinical practice.

It is now clear that treatment with SSRIs can be associated with the development of most forms of sexual dysfunction, again including decreased sexual interest, erectile failure, impaired ejaculation and impaired orgasm. In particular, SSRIs can cause delayed ejaculation in men and anorgasmia in women. This apparent increase is probably the result of more people being treated with SSRIs, and a heightened awareness of the importance of sexual dysfunction, leading doctors to detect and report sexual side effects more frequently.

In the case of fluoxetine, for example, an early review of its tolerability and safety indicated that approximately 5% of patients developed 'treatment-emergent' sexual dysfunction (Stark and Hardison, 1985). Following the launch of fluoxetine, and its widespread clinical use, reports suggested that the incidence of sexual dysfunction was much higher than originally thought. Studies which have employed systematic questioning about the presence of sexual difficulties indicate that sexual dysfunction is present in 34%–75% of patients treated with fluoxetine (Jacobsen, 1992; Balon et al, 1993; Patterson, 1993; Hsu and Shen, 1995) (Table 10).

Fluoxetine and sexual dysfunction:
Apparent increase in incidence of sexual dysfunction probably reflects growing awareness

Study	Year	N	Sexual dysfunction (%)
Stark P, Hardison CD	1985	185	5.0
Herman JB et al	1990	60	8.3
Zajecka J et al	1991	77	7.8
Jacobsen FM	1992	160	34.0
Balon R et al	1993	14	42.9
Patterson WM	1993	60	75.0
Hsu JH, Shen WW	1995	32	43.0

Table 10

The problem of sexual dysfunction is not restricted to fluoxetine, but is also seen with other SSRIs such as sertraline and paroxetine. For example, in a placebo-controlled study of sertraline, the incidence of treatment-emergent male sexual dysfunction was found to be 8.5% at a dose of 50 mg/day, 7.5% at 100 mg/day, and 20.6% at a dose of 200 mg/day (Fabre et al, 1995). Evaluation of sexual dysfunction with paroxetine is somewhat difficult, as although the placebo-adjusted incidence of ejaculatory disturbance is 12.9%, a further 10% of patients experience 'other male genital disorders' which include erectile difficulties, delayed ejaculation, and inhibited orgasm (Medical Economics Data, 1995). The relative incidence of sexual dysfunction with the differing SSRIs is not known.

The effects of nefazodone on sexual function

The antidepressant drug nefazodone has a somewhat unusual mechanism of action, having effects on two complementary sites in serotonergic neurones. It acts on the presynaptic neurone by inhibiting the re-uptake of serotonin, though to a lesser degree than that seen with the selective serotonin re-uptake inhibitors. Nefazodone is also an antagonist at 5-HT_2 receptors on postsynaptic neurones.

This dual mechanism of action of nefazodone may be responsible for the relatively low incidence of SSRI-like side effects seen during clinical trials. For example, nausea and increased agitation appear less common with nefazodone than with SSRIs. It could be that the blockade of postsynaptic receptors reduces the untoward effects of inhibiting the re-uptake of 5-HT into the presynaptic neurones.

The findings of clinical studies show that the incidence of sexual dysfunction with nefazodone is low, in both men and women. Data from the extensive clinical trial database show that there are no significant differences between nefazodone and placebo in the incidence of decreased libido, erectile dysfunction, abnormal ejaculation or anorgasmia reported as a treatment-emergent side effect (Baldwin, 1996). In an overview of placebo-controlled studies involving nefazodone, imipramine, and fluoxetine, there were no significant differences between nefazodone and placebo, whereas both fluoxetine and imipramine were associated with a greater incidence of sexual dysfunction than was seen with placebo (Robinson et al, 1996) (Table 11).

Relative incidence of sexual dysfunction with nefazodone

Treatment emergent sexual dysfunction: all patients				
	Placebo	**Imipramine**	**Fluoxetine**	**Nefazodone**
N	875	367	182	1310
Decreased libido	0.5%	1.6%	2.2%*	0.7%
Psychosexual dysfunction	0%	1.1%*	1.6%*	0.1%
Anorgasmia	0.1%	0.3%	1.1%	0.2%

Treatment emergent sexual dysfunction: men				
	Placebo	**Imipramine**	**Fluoxetine**	**Nefazodone**
N	334	163	61	494
Impotence	1.2%	9.8%*	1.6%	1.4%
Abnormal ejaculation	0%	3.1%*	1.6%	0.2%

* $p < 0.05$ vs. placebo

Source: Robinson (1996)

Table 11

These findings suggest that the incidence of sexual dysfunction with nefazodone is less than that seen with SSRIs. This inference is supported by the results of a comparative trial of the acute treatment of patients suffering from DSM-III-R major depression, which included a systematic evaluation of the effects of nefazodone and sertraline on sexual function, in addition to usual measures of efficacy and tolerability (Feiger et al, 1996) (Figures 2 and 3).

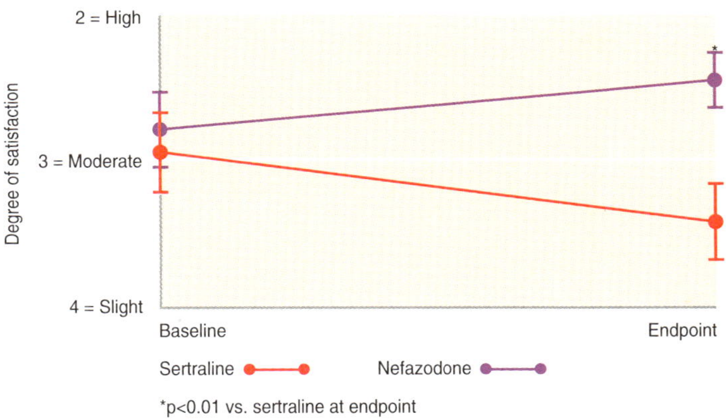

Figure 2
Satisfaction with sexual function (men). Source: Feiger et al (1996).

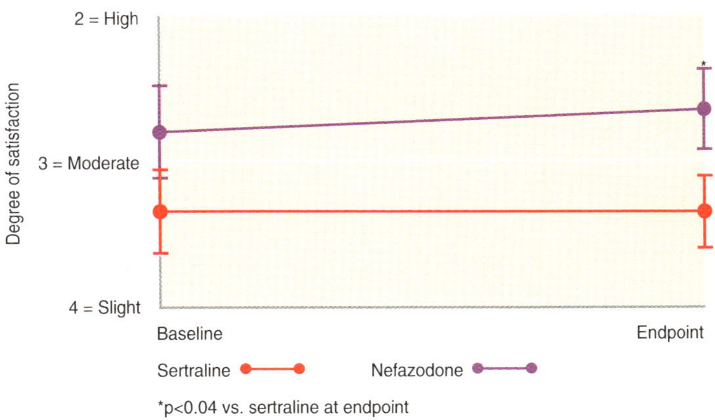

Figure 3
Satisfaction with sexual function (women). Source: Feiger et al (1996).

N.B. *Figures 2 and 3 are sections of graphs where the 'Degree of satisfaction' scale extends from 1 = Complete, to 5 = None at all.*

In this study, nefazodone was found to cause significantly less disturbance of sexual function than sertraline. In women, nefazodone was significantly superior to sertraline on measures of ease in achieving, and satisfaction with, orgasm. In men, treatment with nefazodone was associated with significantly less impairment of sexual enjoyment and satisfaction, and with less difficulty with and delay of ejaculation. By contrast, treatment with sertraline was associated with significantly fewer reports of premature ejaculation, this observation being in line with other findings of delayed ejaculation with sertraline (Feiger et al, 1996).

The relative advantage of nefazodone over sertraline with regard to adverse effects on sexual function and satisfaction have been confirmed by the results of a further study, again in patients suffering from DSM-III-R major depression. In this investigation patients who experienced sexual dysfunction with sertraline were withdrawn from the drug, and then followed up over a 7–10 day placebo washout interval. Those patients who were no longer experiencing sexual dysfunction were then randomized to treatment with either sertraline or nefazodone for a period of 8 weeks. At the end of treatment, 71% of sertraline-treated patients experienced sexual dysfunction, compared to only 30% of patients allocated to treatment with nefazodone (Ferguson et al, 1996) (Figure 4).

Taken together, the findings within the placebo-controlled database and the results of the comparator studies with sertraline indicate that nefazodone has relatively few adverse effects on sexual function. The mechanism underlying this is unclear, but is probably due in part to the blockade of post-synaptic 5-HT_2 receptors, as 5-HT_2 antagonism is found to enhance sexual behaviour in animal models and to improve function in patients experiencing sexual side effects arising from treatment with serotonergic agonists (Baldwin, 1996).

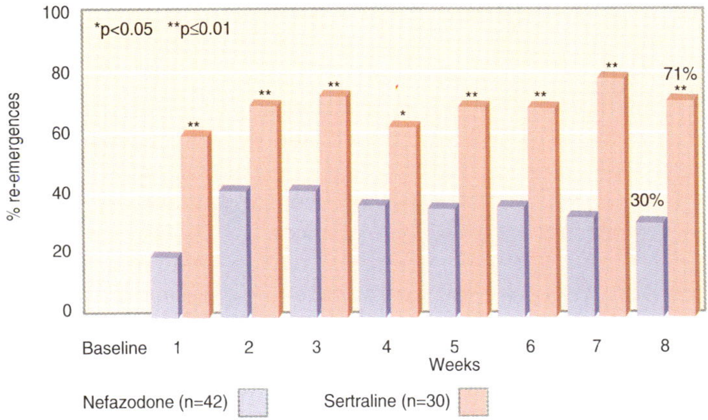

Figure 4
Re-emergence of sexual dysfunction: Difficulty with ejaculation, erection and orgasm in men; orgasmic difficulties, inadequate lubrication and swelling in women. Source: Ferguson et al (1996).

Unusual effects of antidepressant drugs on sexual function

There have been a number of reports of unusual effects of antidepressant drugs on sexual function (Baldwin, 1995). For example, tricyclic antidepressants have been associated with the development of painful ejaculation, which may occur in approximately 20% of men receiving TCAs. Because of the blockade of peripheral sympathetic α-adrenergic receptors, TCAs can interfere with the co-ordinated contractions of smooth muscles involved in sperm transport and therefore cause painful spasm.

Other unusual sexual side effects with antidepressants include penile anaesthesia with fluoxetine, and an unusual syndrome, consisting of yawning and multiple orgasm in the absence of sexual stimulation, which has been described in a few patients treated with clomipramine or fluoxetine.

Trazodone has been associated with the development of priapism (i.e. prolonged painful erection), and with an increase in sexual interest in both men and women. Priapism is an uncommon complication of treatment with trazodone (affecting between 1 : 1,000–10,000 men), and is also seen with other psychotropic drugs, including antipsychotic agents. Patients taking trazodone should be warned of the risk of priapism, and be advised to seek medical attention promptly should it occur. The initial treatment of priapism is medical, and involves irrigation of the corpora cavernosa with either saline or metaraminol (an alpha adrenoceptor agonist). This usually results in venous constriction and subsequent penile detumescence. However, if medical approaches are unsuccessful, surgical procedures may be necessary, and these can unfortunately result in permanent erectile dysfunction.

Adverse effects of other psychotropic drugs on sexual function

Although most antidepressant drugs are effective in relieving anxiety and insomnia in depression, it is not uncommon for depressed patients to be prescribed anxiolytic or hypnotic drugs, in addition to antidepressant medication. Similarly, antipsychotic drugs are sometimes prescribed as concomitant treatments in depressed patients, usually when depression is accompanied by marked agitation or psychosis. Furthermore, long-term treatment of patients with bipolar affective disorder or recurrent unipolar depression can involve the use of lithium and anticonvulsant drugs. Unfortunately, most of these other psychotropic drugs can also be associated with the development of sexual dysfunction (Baldwin, 1995).

Antipsychotic (neuroleptic) drugs

Many patients taking antipsychotic drugs complain of sexual problems, which may be the reason given for non-compliance with treatment. The most common sexual complaints in men are of erectile dysfunction, delayed orgasm and orgasm without ejaculation. Women treated with antipsychotic drugs commonly describe menstrual irregularities, loss of sexual interest, reduced fertility and galactorrhoea (Barnes and Harvey, 1993).

In general, the sexual side effects of antipsychotic drugs are largely dose related. The pathophysiological mechanisms include the blockade of dopamine receptors which is common to all conventional neuroleptics, and the elevation of serum prolactin levels. When compared to conventional antipsychotic drugs, the 'atypical' neuroleptic compound clozapine seems to be associated with a lower incidence of sexual side effects, perhaps due to the relatively low occupancy of dopamine D-2 receptors, or to the reduced risk of causing hyperprolactinaemia.

Hyperprolactinaemia increases the incidence of sexual side effects in men and women. The loss of sexual interest that is common in patients with hyperprolactinaemia can be improved by the use of dopamine agonists such as bromocriptine, but use of these drugs can be hazardous, as they may worsen psychosis.

Benzodiazepines

The sexual side effects of benzodiazepine hypnotics and anxiolytics have not been investigated extensively. Although originally recommended in the management of patients with sexual dysfunction, there seems little doubt that benzodiazepines can reduce sexual desire and performance. In a placebo-controlled study in women volunteers, single doses of diazepam were found to reduce arousability and vaginal lubrication, and significantly delay orgasm (Riley and Riley, 1986). Furthermore, in a series of case reports, benzodiazepines have also been associated with decreased sexual interest, erectile dysfunction and anorgasmia.

Buspirone

As buspirone is a 5-HT agonist, it might be expected to inhibit sexual desire. However, it is fairly specific for the 5-HT_{1a} receptor, and has been found to stimulate male sexual behaviour in experimental animals. A single open study of the effects of buspirone in patients with an anxiety state and sexual dysfunction suggested that it had beneficial effects on sexual interest and function. Buspirone has been advocated as an adjunctive agent in the management of sexual dysfunction arising from treatment with antidepressant drugs (Norden, 1995).

Lithium

Although a number of reports have linked the use of lithium salts to the development of sexual dysfunction, there is no consistent pattern to the adverse events. A recent study indicated that patients treated with benzodiazepines and lithium in combination had a higher rate of sexual dysfunction, compared to patients treated with lithium alone. Sexual problems with lithium do not appear to be related to serum levels.

Anticonvulsant drugs

Anticonvulsant drugs are being used more frequently in psychiatric practice, both in the prophylaxis of bipolar affective disorder, and as adjuvant treatments in patients with affective illness or schizophrenia. Although many anticonvulsant drugs have been reported to have adverse effects on normal sexual function, it should be remembered that epilepsy is itself probably associated with a reduction in sexual interest and activity. There is some evidence to show that erectile dysfunction in male epileptic patients improves when adequate seizure control has been achieved (Peet and Gillow, 1993).

The actions of anticonvulsant drugs on sexual function probably arise from a combination of differing mechanisms. Firstly, many anticonvulsants induce the hepatic enzymes that are responsible for the metabolism of steroid hormones. Secondly, certain drugs induce the production of sex-hormone-binding globulin, and can lower the levels of free testosterone.

When compared to other anticonvulsant drugs, carbamazepine may have fewer effects on the levels of testosterone, which could account for the relative scarcity of adverse effects on sexual function. Sodium valproate does not alter the metabolism of sex hormones, and should be associated with a low incidence of sexual side effects.

Sexual side effects of drugs used to treat physical illness

Clearly, many psychotropic drugs can have adverse effects on sexual function. This is also the case with many other classes of prescribed medication, although the quality of information regarding sexual side effects varies widely (Table 12). The most reliable data are obtained during the course of double-blind placebo-controlled trials, but these are costly and difficult

Drugs used to treat physical illness that can have adverse effects on sexual function

Class	Example
Antihypertensives	Thiazide diuretics, beta-blockers
Anticonvulsants	Carbamazepine
Antihistamines	Cimetidine
Cytotoxic agents	Vinblastine, methotrexate
Lipid-lowering agents	Clofibrate
Opiate analgesics	Diamorphine
Others	Digoxin, disulfiram

Sources: Huws (1993); Peet and Gillow (1993)

Table 12

to perform, and consequently the evaluation of adverse effects tends to rely on other, less satisfactory, methods such as case series or single case reports (Baldwin, 1995).

The prevalence of sexual problems increases with age and is higher in populations with medical or psychiatric illness. Sexual dysfunction which may appear to be drug related must be assessed against this increased background prevalence. As well as direct effects on sexual health, many medical conditions have non-specific effects on sexual function, for example problems due to anxiety resulting from the process of medical diagnosis and treatment. By contrast, sexual dysfunction associated with a particular illness can be improved by successful drug treatment of that illness (Peet and Gillow, 1993).

Depressive illness is associated with increased morbidity for a number of physical conditions, including cardiovascular disease, gastrointestinal problems and neurological disorders. Many depressed patients also have co-morbid physical health problems. As described above, many medical conditions are associated with the development of sexual dysfunction. The assessment of sexual difficulties in a depressed patient should therefore include not only an evaluation of the presence and severity of any co-morbid somatic illness but also a consideration of any possible sexual side effects of concomitant treatment (Wise, 1992).

Management of sexual dysfunction

Psychological approaches to sexual dysfunction

Psychological factors play an extremely important part in the sexual response, and mood is an essential determinant of sexual function. Low mood with associated low self-esteem will affect an individual's attractiveness and sense of being desired. Furthermore, depression can cause or contribute to relationship difficulties and thus affect a couple's sexual relationship. The management of such problems is often complex and multifaceted, involving a combination of psychological and pharmacological approaches.

Depressed patients who are troubled by sexual dysfunction can often be helped by some of the general psychological approaches to the management of people with sexual difficulties. These approaches aim to reduce anxiety and foster feelings of security. By establishing better patterns of communication between partners, any sense of failure or resentment can often be reduced (Bancroft, 1989).

Psychological approaches may be either specifically targeted at the particular sexual problems, or more broadly directed at the overall relationship. Those which have been found successful include:

- Counselling and brief supportive psychotherapy
- Couple therapy
- Individual therapy
- Group therapy

Studies of the outcome of psychological interventions have revealed varying degrees of success. A survey of sex therapists suggests that up to 52% of men suffering from psychogenic erectile dysfunction can be helped by these approaches (Kilman et al, 1986), particularly when this dysfunction is 'secondary' i.e., when at least one successful attempt at sexual intercourse has occurred (Lobitz and Baker, 1979).

Counselling and brief supportive psychotherapy

This can be carried out effectively and cheaply in the setting of an outpatient clinic. Issues to be dealt with include ignorance, misunderstanding, guilt and anxiety. Often all that is required is the provision of limited information, reassurance, permission and the encouragement and facilitation of better communication between the couple.

Couple therapy

This is based largely on behavioural theories, but also incorporates some educational and psychodynamic components. The broad objective is to develop a stable relationship in which normal sexual responses can take place, and from which pleasure can be derived. This can be effective in tackling many forms of sexual dysfunction, including the anorgasmia encountered in some depressed patients.

In essence, 'homework' is set by the therapist, involving a system of graded touching, termed 'sensate focus'. At first, this sets strict limits on the encounter, and usually excludes genital touching and sexual intercourse. Other problems, such as poor communication, ignorance and relationship difficulties, can be tackled by the psychotherapist as they are encountered. In addition, cognitive, psychodynamic and behavioural techniques may be employed as necessary.

Individual therapy

This is usually undertaken when the patient has no current partner, or where a partner is unwilling to participate in treatment. Essentially, it involves the same range of approaches as that for couple therapy.

Group therapy

This is more common in the USA than in Europe. It is usually conducted as single sex groups, where members of the group have similar sexual problems. Again, many approaches to treatment can be employed, although most groups were psychoanalytically orientated until recent years.

People with sexual problems can sometimes be helped by involvement in patient support organisations. Although self-help groups for sexual problems are relatively popular in the USA, they have not become established in the UK. The self-help organisation *Us Too* was set up in the USA by a patient whose surgery for cancer of the prostate gland had rendered him impotent (Kaps, 1994).

In addition to these individual, couple and group psychotherapeutic approaches, a number of specific behavioural techniques have been developed to improve particular aspects of sexual performance. These include intermittent penetration for men with erectile failure, and guided masturbation for delayed ejaculation or anorgasmia (Bancroft, 1989).

Pharmacological approaches to sexual dysfunction

The psychological and behavioural strategies that are used in the management of patients with sexual dysfunction can be complemented by a range of pharmacological approaches (Table 13).

Pharmacological management of sexual dysfunction
Continuation of current treatment
Delayed dosing
Reduction in dosage
Withdrawal of medication
'Drug holidays'
Adjunctive agents
Substitution with alternative treatment
Sources: Segraves (1993); Gitlin (1994); Baldwin (1995)

Table 13

Clearly, treatment strategies should be tailored to the individual patient, taking into account the benefits and risks of each approach. However the emergence of sexual dysfunction is an important cause of non-compliance in depressed patients treated with antidepressants. Effective management of sexual problems should be expected to result in improved adherence to treatment, and therefore enhance the long-term clinical outcome (Balon et al, 1993).

Expectant management

Certain aspects of sexual dysfunction may remit, simply with the passage of time. The rate of accommodation to the sexual side effects of antidepressant drugs is not known. Remission has been reported in some patients taking MAOIs and SSRIs, but successful changes in sexual technique may give a misleading impression that an adverse effect has spontaneously resolved (Baldwin, 1995).

Delayed dosing

Some patients with drug-induced sexual dysfunction may note improvements simply by postponing taking their medication until after sexual intercourse (Olivera, 1994). This approach allows them to continue with the same drug at the same dose, but is only likely to be helpful with antidepressant drugs that have a short half-life. Furthermore some patients — and their partners — may feel unsettled by the thought of taking an antidepressant after sexual activity!

Reduction in dosage

Adverse effects on sexual function may be more common with higher doses of medication. For example, sexual dysfunction has been reported as being more common with higher doses of a range of antidepressant drugs, including imipramine, clomipramine, desipramine, maprotiline, protriptyline and fluoxetine. However, many patients develop sexual problems, even whilst taking low doses of antidepressant drugs. A reduction in dose is often possible — with fluoxetine, for example, optimal efficacy in depression is often seen with a daily dose of 20 mg (or less) but higher doses are often used in clinical practice.

Withdrawal of medication

When distressing sexual dysfunction persists even after allowing for the passage of time and a reduction in dose, withdrawal of treatment may be necessary. In most cases, withdrawal of medication leads to the recovery of sexual function within a few days. With fluoxetine, resolution takes rather longer, probably because of the extended half-life of the drug and its principal metabolite. Of course, withdrawal of medication runs the risk of precipitating a relapse of depression.

'Drug holidays'

Recently, 'drug holidays' have been advocated in the management of patients with sexual dysfunction induced by SSRIs (Rothschild, 1995) (Table 14). Treatment is interrupted briefly, 1–2 days before anticipated sexual activity. Beneficial effects on sexual function have been seen in patients treated with paroxetine and sertraline, though not with fluoxetine (presumably because of its long half-life). Although encouraging, these findings are somewhat preliminary, as the published studies were of an 'open' design, and involved only small numbers of patients. Furthermore, it is likely that many patients would find this approach aesthetically unacceptable.

Drug holidays

Percentage of patients who reported 'much' or 'very much' improved sexual function. Improvement noted in at least 2 of 4 weekends.

	Fluoxetine	Paroxetine	Sertraline
N	10	10	10
Mean daily dose	24 mg	26 mg	60 mg
Orgasm function	10%	50%	60%
Sexual satisfaction	0%	50%	50%
Libido	0%	50%	50%

Source: Rothschild (1995)

Table 14

Treatment substitution

A number of reports have described the effect of switching from one drug to another, in an attempt to reduce the incidence or severity of sexual dysfunction. There have been case reports of successful drug substitutions that include desipramine for imipramine and clomipramine, imipramine for amoxapine, nortriptyline for imipramine and doxepin, and bupropion for numerous antidepressants. Recent studies have suggested that nefazodone is a useful and appropriate alternative in patients who develop sexual dysfunction with sertraline, and probably with other SSRIs (Ferguson et al, 1996). It is unclear whether greater benefit arises from substituting with a drug from the same class of antidepressant drug, or whether it is more helpful to choose a drug from a different class of compound.

Adjunctive treatments

Further pharmacological strategies in the management of drug-induced sexual dysfunction include the use of so-called adjunctive or adjuvant compounds (Table 15) (Baldwin, 1996).

Adjunctive treatments

Class	Example
Serotonin antagonists	Cyproheptadine, mianserin
5-HT$_{1a}$ partial agonists	Buspirone
Adrenergic antagonists	Yohimbine, fluparoxan
Cholinergic agonists	Neostigmine, bethanechol
Dopamine agonists	Amantadine, dextroamphetamine, pemoline

Sources: Segraves (1989); Gitlin (1994); Baldwin (1995)

Table 15

Cyproheptadine, an antagonist at serotonin and histamine receptors, has been found to be useful in the management of anorgasmia associated with TCAs, MAOIs, and SSRIs. Typically, 2–16 mg of cyproheptadine are taken 1–2 hours prior to anticipated sexual activity. Unfortunately, use of cyproheptadine can sometimes result in the reversal of the therapeutic effects of antidepressants (Feder, 1991; Hollander et al, 1992).

The antidepressant drug **mianserin** acts as an antagonist, both at 5-HT$_2$ and 5-HT$_3$ receptors and at α-2 adrenoceptors. As the 5-HT$_2$ antagonist properties of mianserin have been thought responsible for its efficacy in managing the akathisia occasionally seen with SSRIs (Poyurovsky et al, 1995), it should at least in theory be of some value in reversing SSRI-induced anorgasmia. However, mianserin has itself been linked to the development of sexual dysfunction (Kowalski et al, 1985).

As mentioned earlier, **buspirone** appears to have fewer adverse effects on sexual function than other anxiolytic drugs. It has been used in the management of sexual dysfunction in patients treated with SSRIs. Although the mechanism of action of these beneficial properties is unclear, it probably involves inhibition of central serotonergic neurotransmission, arising from effects on pre-synaptic 5-HT$_{1a}$ autoreceptors.

The adrenergic **alpha-2 antagonists** yohimbine and fluparoxan may have beneficial effects in relieving erectile dysfunction. The mechanism of action is not fully understood, but may involve both a central effect in enhancing sexual interest, and a peripheral effect on alpha-2 receptors within the corpora cavernosa of the penis. Two approaches to treatment with yohimbine have been advocated — either a regular daily dose of 5.4 mg three times daily, or a dose of 5.4–16.2 mg taken

2–4 hours before sex. The side effects of yohimbine include excessive perspiration, urinary frequency, anxiety, insomnia and fatigue.

Cholinergic agonists such as neostigmine and bethanechol have been reported to reverse the loss of sexual desire associated with amitriptyline, and anorgasmia linked to other TCAs. Treatment with bethanechol involves either a regular daily dose of 30–100 mg, or the use of 10–40 mg shortly before sexual intercourse. The side effects of bethanechol include diarrhoea, cramps and excessive perspiration.

Finally, **dopamine agonists** such as amantadine, dextroamphetamine and pemoline have been found to be helpful in reversing anorgasmia associated with the use of fluoxetine, sertraline and phenelzine. The mechanism of this effect is unclear, but probably involves either direct dopaminergic effects in increasing libido and facilitating ejaculation, or indirect actions through reversing the inhibition of dopaminergic transmission that is seen with some serotonergic compounds.

Unfortunately, there have been few double-blind placebo-controlled trials of these drugs in depressed patients. Most of the evidence of benefit comes from anecdotal case reports. In the absence of convincing evidence, doctors should be cautious when using unfamiliar treatments, particularly when they carry the risk of reversing the beneficial effects of antidepressant drugs.

Physical treatments of sexual dysfunction

The physical treatments of sexual dysfunction are directed mainly toward the man with erectile failure, usually secondary to an underlying chronic illness such as diabetes or multiple sclerosis. They are not so appropriate in those whose sexual dysfunction is psychologically based or secondary to the use of psychotropic medication as these problems are likely to respond to psychotherapeutic and pharmacological strategies. The physical treatments for men with organically determined sexual dysfunction differ in their technique, efficacy and acceptability (Kirby, 1994) (Table 16).

Physical treatments for erectile dysfunction	
Intracavernosal pharmacotherapy	Papaverine Alprostadil
Surgical treatments	Revascularization surgery Venous leak correction
Use of a vacuum device	
Penile prostheses	
	Source: Dawson and Whitfield (1996)

Table 16

Intracavernosal pharmacotherapy

The possibility of inducing an erection by injection of papaverine (a smooth muscle relaxant) into the corpora cavernosa was first discovered in the early 1980s. It provided an effective treatment for many patients with neurogenic or psychogenic impotence and could be administered by the patient when erection was required. More recently alprostadil (prostaglandin E1) by intracavernosal injection has been demonstrated to be efficacious in the treatment of erectile failure and is probably safer than papaverine, having a reduced incidence of prolonged erection. Alprostadil has the added benefit of being licensed in the UK for the treatment of erectile failure (Anonymous, 1995).

The main side effect of intracavernosal injections is prolonged erection or priapism and patients are advised to seek medical help should their erection be maintained for more than four hours. Pain and fibrosis at the site of injection may also occur. A dropout rate of 50% has been reported, couples usually stating inconvenience or difficulty with the technique as reasons for ceasing its use.

Surgical treatments

These may be indicated for patients with specific problems such as peripheral vascular disease where some success has been reported in younger patients undergoing revascularization surgery. Excision and ligation of the deep dorsal vein has been demonstrated as effective in a few patients with venous leakage causing erectile failure.

Use of a vacuum device

These have been used either as a first line treatment, especially in the older or more physically unwell patient or in those who have failed to respond to intracavernosal injection. The technique is non-invasive, requiring the patient to place the penis into a cylindrical vacuum device. A hand or battery operated pump draws air out, thereby creating a vacuum which draws blood into the penis. A constriction ring is then placed over the base of the penis which maintains the erection. Complications are minimal but patients may experience bruising, discomfort and sometimes difficulty in ejaculating. Although 70% of men report an erection sufficient for intercourse, many complain that the result is far from satisfactory.

Penile prosthesis

This requires surgical insertion, under general anaesthesia, of a semi-rigid or inflatable device — the latter being more commonly in use. This technique is used only where intracavernosal therapy and vacuum devices have failed, and the prostheses are expensive. Infection is the most serious complication necessitating removal of the device.

The importance of correct investigation and assessment cannot be overemphasized. A multidisciplinary approach to the management of erectile dysfunction is ideal. Those patients with interpersonal or relationship difficulties are unlikely to find that these physical techniques for the management of erectile impotence do anything to improve their overall sexual function.

Treatment of premature ejaculation

Premature ejaculation is a common but under-reported disorder. In an analysis of 22 surveys of the general population, up to 35% of men had experienced premature ejaculation (Nathan, 1986). Although rather more common than erectile failure, fewer patients present for treatment, usually consulting general practitioners rather than hospital specialists (Shahar et al, 1991).

Some patients are helped by explanation and reassurance alone, or by the knowledge that premature ejaculation often resolves with increasing experience and confidence in sexual relationships. Others will need to be helped by instruction in behavioural approaches, designed to gain greater control of arousal and ejaculation. These include the 'start-stop' technique and the 'squeeze technique' (for further details, see Bancroft, 1989).

When premature ejaculation persists despite these simple psychological and behavioural approaches, some patients benefit from treatment with antidepressant drugs. As might be expected from their association with the adverse effect of delayed ejaculation, both clomipramine and the SSRIs have been evaluated in uncontrolled studies in men with persistent troublesome premature ejaculation.

Clomipramine has been found beneficial in two double-blind placebo-controlled studies, doses of 25–50 mg being associated with longer ejaculatory delay, greater emotional satisfaction, and improvements in partner orgasmic attainment (Segraves, 1993; Althof et al, 1995). Both paroxetine and sertraline have been evaluated in placebo-controlled studies, and again both drugs have been found helpful (Waldinger et al, 1994; Mendels et al, 1995). These investigations used rather high doses of medication (paroxetine 40 mg/day; sertraline 200 mg/day), and the efficacy of lower daily doses, or intermittent dosing is not established.

Conclusions

As stated in the introduction, adequate sexual expression is an essential component of human relationships, and may promote quality of life and a sense of physical, psychological and social well-being. Unfortunately, depressive illness is associated with a range of impairments of sexual function and satisfaction, and the presence of these problems can worsen a quality of life that is already reduced by the effects of depression.

The existing established antidepressant drugs are far from ideal. Most classes of antidepressant drug can have adverse effects on sexual function. The exact incidence of sexual dysfunction with antidepressants is not known. However, it is likely to be greater than presently thought because of factors such as a certain degree of embarrassment, both in patients and doctors, when discussing sexual problems. Disturbances of sexual interest and performance will only be detected in a reliable fashion when doctors learn to make systematic enquiries during the course of the standard clinical interview.

The growing awareness of the adverse effects of many antidepressants on sexual function should lead to a re-evaluation of earlier claims for the good tolerability of many of the newer drugs. There is a clear need for further adequately designed controlled investigations of the effects of antidepressants on sexual function, so that the tolerability of differing drugs can be assessed in a reliable and replicable fashion.

But more than research is required. At present, doctors gain most of their professional knowledge of sexual function and health by a somewhat haphazard process. Little time and space is made available for teaching medical students about sexual matters, and this paucity of teaching continues into the postgraduate years. Teaching and training in human sexuality should become more fully incorporated into both undergraduate and postgraduate medical education. The resulting increased awareness of the importance of sexual health should then lead to greater attention by doctors to all aspects of the quality of life of their patients.

References

Althof SE, Levine SB, Corty W et al (1995) A double-blind crossover trial of clomipramine for rapid ejaculation in 15 couples. *Journal of Clinical Psychiatry* **56**: 402–7.

American Psychiatric Association (1994) *Diagnostic and Statistical Manual of Mental Disorders* (4th edn). Washington DC: *American Psychiatric Association*.

Anonymous (1995) Alprostadil for erectile impotence. *Drugs and Therapeutics Bulletin* **33**: 61–2.

Athanasiou R, Shaver P, Travis C (1970) Sex. *Psychology Today* **4**: 39–52.

Baldwin DS (1995) Psychotropic drugs and sexual dysfunction. *International Review of Psychiatry* **7**: 261–73.

Baldwin DS (1996) Depression and sexual function. *Journal of Psychopharmacology* **10** (Suppl.): 30–34.

Balon R, Yeragani VK, Pohl R and Ramesh C (1993) Sexual dysfunction during antidepressant treatment. *Journal of Clinical Psychiatry* **54**: 209–12.

Bancroft J (1989) *Human Sexuality and its Problems*, (2nd edn). Edinburgh: Churchill Livingston.

Barnes TRE and Harvey CA (1993) Psychiatric drugs and sexuality. In Riley A, Peet M, Wilson C (eds) *Sexual Pharmacology*. Oxford: Oxford Medical Publications, pp 176–96.

Crowe M (1995) Couple therapy and sexual dysfunction. *International Review of Psychiatry* **7**: 195–204.

Dawson C and Whitfield H (eds) (1996) *ABC of Urology*. London: British Medical Association Publications.

Ende J, Rockwell S, Glasgow M (1984) The sexual history in general medicine practice. *Archives of Internal Medicine* **144**: 558–61.

Fabre LF, Abuzzahab FS, Amin M et al (1995) Sertraline safety and efficacy in major depression: a double-blind fixed-dose comparison with placebo. *Biological Psychiatry* **38**: 592–602.

Fagan PJ, Schmidt CW Jr, Wise TN et al (1985) Sexual dysfunction and dual psychiatric diagnoses. *Comprehensive Psychiatry* **29**: 278–84.

Feder R (1991) Reversal of antidepressant activity of fluoxetine by cyproheptadine in three patients. *Journal of Clinical Psychiatry* **52**: 163.

Feiger A, Kiev A, Shrivastava R et al (1996) Nefazodone versus sertraline in outpatients with major depression : focus on efficacy, tolerability, and effects on sexual function and satisfaction. *Journal of Clinical Psychiatry* **57** (Suppl. 2) 53–62.

Ferguson JM, Shrivastava R, Stahl SM et al (1996) *Effects of double-blind treatment with nefazodone and sertraline on re-emergence of sexual dysfunction in depressed patients NR358*. Presented at the American Psychiatric Association Annual Meeting, May 4–9, 1996, New York, NY, USA.

Frank E, Anderson C, Rubinstein D (1978) Frequency of sexual dysfunction in 'normal' couples. *New England Journal of Medicine* **299**: 111–15.

Frenken J and Van Tol P (1987) Sexual problems in gynaecological practice. *Journal of Psychosomatic Obstetrics and Gynaecology* **6**: 143–55.

Gitlin MJ (1994) Psychotropic medications and their effects on sexual function: diagnosis, biology, and treatment approaches. *Journal of Clinical Psychiatry* **55**: 406–13.

Golombok S, Rust J, Pickard C (1984) Sexual problems encountered in general practice. *British Journal of Sexual Medicine* **11**: 210–12.

Harrison WM, Rabkin JG, Ehrhardt AA, Stewart JW, McGrath PJ, Ross D, Quitkin FM (1986) Effects of antidepressant medication on sexual function: a controlled study. *Journal of Clinical Psychopharmacology* **6**: 144–49.

Herman JB, Brotman AW, Pollack E et al (1990) Fluoxetine — induced sexual dysfunction. *Journal of Clinical Psychiatry* **51**: 25–27.

Hollander ER, Mullen LS, Carrasco JL et al (1992) Symptom relapse in bulimia nervosa and obsessive compulsive disorders after treatment with serotonin antagonists. *Journal of Clinical Psychiatry* **53**: 207–9.

Hsu JH and Shen WW (1995) Male sexual side effects associated with antidepressants: a descriptive study of 32 patients. *International Journal of Psychiatry and Medicine* **25**: 191–201.

Huws R (1993) Antihypertensive medication and sexual problems. In: *Sexual Pharmacology* A Riley, M Peet, C Wilson. pp 146–58. Oxford: Oxford Medical Publications.

Huws R and Sampson G (1993) Recreational drugs and sexuality. In Riley A, Peet M, Wilson C (eds) *Sexual Pharmacology*. Oxford: Oxford Medical Publications. pp 197–210.

Jacobsen FM (1992) Fluoxetine-induced sexual dysfunction and an open trial of yohimbine. *Journal of Clinical Psychiatry* **53**: 119–22.

Kaps EC (1994) The role of the support group 'Us Too'. *Cancer* **74**: 2188–89.

Kilman PR, Boland JP, Norton SP et al (1986) Perspectives of sex therapy outcome: a survey of AASECT providers. *Journal of Sex and Marital Therapy* **12**: 116–38.

Kirby RS (1994) Impotence: diagnosis and management of male erectile dysfunction. *British Medical Journal* **308**: 957–60.

Kivela S-L and Pahkala K (1988) Symptoms of depression in aged Finns. *International Journal of Social Psychiatry* **34**: 274–84.

Klassen AD and Wilsnack SC (1986) Sexual experience and drinking among women in a US national survey. *Archives of Sexual Behaviour* **15**: 363–92.

Kockott G and Pfeiffer W (1996) Sexual disorders in non-acute psychiatric out-patients. *Comprehensive Psychiatry* **37**: 56–61.

Kowalski A, Stanley RP, Dennerstein L et al (1985) The sexual side effects of antidepressant medication: a double-blind comparison of two antidepressants in a non-psychiatric population. *British Journal of Psychiatry* **147**: 413–18.

Levine SB and Yost MA (1976) Frequency of sexual dysfunction in a general gynaecological clinic: an epidemiological approach. *Archives of Sexual Behaviour* **5**: 229–38.

Lobitz WC and Baker EL (1979) Group treatment of secondary erectile dysfunction. *Journal of Sex and Marital Therapy* **8**: 127–38.

Mandell W and Miller CM (1983) Male sexual dysfunction as related to alcohol consumption: a pilot study. *Alcohol Clinical and Experimental Research* **7**: 65–9.

Matthew RJ and Weinman ML (1982) Sexual dysfunction in depression. *Archives of Sexual Behaviour* **11**: 323–28.

Medical Economics Data (1995) Paxil (paroxetine hydrochloride). In: *Physicians Desk Reference*, New Jersey: Medical Economics Data Production Company, pp 239–95.

Mendels J, Camera A, Sikes C (1995) Sertraline treatment for premature ejaculation. *Journal of Clinical Psychopharmacology* **15**: 341–46.

Monteiro WO, Norshirvani HF, Marks IM et al (1987) Anorgasmia from clomipramine in obsessive compulsive disorder: a controlled trial. *British Journal of Psychiatry* **151**: 107–12.

MORI (1995) *Depression*. Research study conducted for LMB Public Relations on behalf of Bristol-Myers Squibb. London: MORI.

Nathan SG (1986) The epidemiology of DSM-III psychosexual dysfunctions. *Journal of Sex and Marital Therapy* **12**: 267–82.

Norden MJ (1995) Buspirone treatment of sexual dysfunction associated with selective serotonin reuptake inhibitors. *Depression* **2**: 109–12.

Olivera AA (1994) Sexual dysfunction due to clomipramine and sertraline: non-pharmacological resolution. *Journal of Sex Education and Therapy* **20**: 119–20.

Patterson WM (1993) Fluoxetine-induced sexual dysfunction. *Journal of Clinical Psychiatry* **54**: 71.

Peet M and Gillow J (1993) The effect on sexual function of anticonvulsant, antiparkinsonian and other miscellaneous drugs. In: (eds A Riley, M Peet, C Wilson) *Sexual Pharmacology*. Oxford Medical Publications, pp 159–75 Oxford.

Philipp M, Kohnen R, Benkert O (1993) A comparison study of moclobemide and doxepin in major depression with special reference to effects on sexual dysfunction. *International Clinical Psychopharmacology* **7**: 123–32.

Potts S and Bhugra D (1995) Classification of sexual disorders. *International Review of Psychiatry* **7 (2)**: 167–74.

Poyurovsky M and Weizman A (1995) Beneficial effect of low-dose mianserin on fluoxamine-induced akathisia in an OCD patient. *International Clinical Psychopharmacology* **10**: 111–14.

Riley AJ and Riley EJ (1986) The effects of single dose diazepam on female sexual response induced by masturbation. *Journal of Sex and Marital Therapy* **1**: 49–54.

Riley A, Peet M, Wilson C, editors (1993) *Sexual Pharmacology*. Oxford: Oxford Medical Publications.

Robinson DS, Roberts DL, Smith JM et al (1996) The safety profile of nefazodone. *Journal of Clinical Psychiatry* **57** (Suppl.): 31–8.

Rothschild AJ (1995) Selective serotonin re-uptake inhibitor-induced sexual dysfunction: efficacy of a drug holiday. *American Journal of Psychiatry* **152**: 1514–16.

Schreiner-Engel P and Schiavi RC (1986) Lifetime psychopathology in individuals with low sexual desire. *Journal of Nervous and Mental Disease* **174**: 646–51.

Schiavi RC (1992) Interview, psychometric and psychophysiologic strategies to assess sexual disorder aetiology. *Journal of Clinical Psychiatry* **10**: 19–26.

Segraves RT (1989) Effect of psychotropic drugs on human erection and ejaculation. *Archives of General Psychiatry* **46**: 275–84.

Segraves RT (1993) Treatment-emergent sexual dysfunction in affective disorder: a review and management strategies. *Journal of Clinical Psychiatry* **11**: 57–60.

Shahar E, Leder J, Herz MJ (1991) The use of a self-report questionnaire to assess the frequency of sexual dysfunction in family practice clinics. *Family Practice* **8**: 206–12.

Shen WW and Sata LS (1983) Inhibited female orgasm resulting from psychotropic drugs: a clinical review. *Journal of Reproductive Medicine* **2**: 497–99.

Shen WW and Sata LS (1990) Inhibited female orgasm resulting from psychotropic drugs: a five-year update. *Journal of Reproductive Medcine* **35**: 11–14.

Slag M, Morley JE, Elson MK et al (1983) Impotence in medical outpatient clinics. *Journal of the American Medical Association* **249**: 1736–40.

Spitzer RL, Endicott J, Robins E (1978) Research diagnostic criteria: rationale and reliability. *Archives of General Psychiatry* **35**: 773–82.

Stark P and Hardison CD (1985) A review of multicenter controlled studies of fluoxetine versus imipramine and placebo in outpatients with major depressive disorder. *Journal of Clinical Psychiatry* **46**: 53–8.

Swan M and Wilson MJ (1979) Sexual and marital problems in a psychiatric outpatient population. *British Journal of Psychiatry* **135**: 310–14.

Wadsworth J and Johnson AM (1994) Physical health and sexual behaviour. In: *Sexual Behaviour in Britain. The National Survey of Sexual Attitudes and Lifestyles* (eds K Wellings, J Field, AM Johnson, J Wadsworth) pp 275–324. London: Penguin.

Waldinger MD, Hengeveld MW, Zwinderman AH (1994) Paroxetine treatment of premature ejaculation: a double-blind randomized placebo controlled study. *American Journal of Psychiatry* **151**: 1377–79.

Webster L (1996) Sexual problems. *Medicine* **24 (3)**: 66–68.

Wellings K, Field J, Johnson AM , Wadsworth J, editors (1994) *Sexual Behaviour in Britain. The National Survey of Sexual Attitudes and Lifestyles*. London: Penguin.

Wesson PR (1982) Cocaine use by masseuses. *Journal of Psychoactive Drugs* **14**: 75–6.

Whalley LJ (1978) Sexual adjustments of male alcoholics. *Acta Psychiatrica Scandinavica* **58**: 281–98.

Wilson CA (1993) Pharmacological targets for the control of male and female sexual behaviour. In: Riley A, Peet M, Wilson C (eds) *Sexual Pharmacology*, Oxford: Oxford Medical Publications, pp 1–58.

Wise TN (1992) A model for the assessment of sexual dysfunction aetiology. *Journal of Clinical Psychiatry* **10**: 11–18.

World Health Organisation (1992) *The ICD-10 Classification of Mental and Behavioural Disorders: Clinical Descriptions and Diagnostic Guidelines*. Geneva: World Health Organisation.

Zajecka J, Fawcett J, Schaff F et al (1991) The role of serotonin in sexual dysfunction: fluoxetine — associated orgasm dysfunction. *Journal of Clinical Psychiatry* **52**: 66–68.

Further Reading

John Bancroft (1989) *Human Sexuality and its Problems,* second edition. Churchill Livingston, Edinburgh.
The definitive textbook.

Dinesh Bhugra and Padmal de Silva (1995) Psychosexual Medicine. *International Review of Psychiatry* **7 (2)**.
Single-subject issue, containing papers of historical and cultural interest.

Chris Dawson and Hugh Whitfield (eds) (1996) *ABC of Urology.* British Medical Association Publications, London.
Contains a clear and concise review of aspects of sexual dysfunction.

Alan Riley, Malcolm Peet and Catherine Wilson (eds) (1993) *Sexual Pharmacology.* Oxford Medical Publications, Oxford.
Probably of greatest interest to psychopharmacologists.

Kaye Wellings, Julia Field, Anne M Johnson, Jane Wadsworth (1994) *Sexual Behaviour in Britain. The National Survey of Sexual Attitudes and Lifestyles.* Penguin, London.
Design and results of the first authoritative survey of sexual behaviour in Britain.

Index

Page numbers in italic refer to the illustrations

PATIENT INFORMATION

A patient leaflet on sexual function and depression plus a patient sexual function self-assessment questionnaire are available from:

Depression Alliance
PO Box 1022
London SE1 7QB
Tel: 0171-721 7672 (answerphone only)